Positive Affirmations for Black Women to Increase Confidence and Self-Love

Written for BIPOC Women with a Focus on Motivation, Leadership, Healing, Growth, Health, Money, and Success

Kayla Holder

Copyright 2021 Kayla Holder

All Rights Reserved.

No portion of this book may be reproduced in any form without permission from the publisher, except as permitted by U.S. copyright law.

This book makes no claims or promises to the reader.

Table of Contents

INTRODUCTION --- 7

AFFIRMATIONS --- 9

JOURNAL --- 18

INTRODUCTION

These affirmations speak to the black woman you currently are and are going to become. As you read through them, I encourage you to pause and reflect on each one - particularly focusing on how they make you feel. As you absorb these affirmations, I suggest you choose your favorites, write them down, and speak them over yourself as often as you need. I have included blank journaling pages in the back of the book so you can record any thoughts you have as you reflect on yourself as a black woman journeying towards increased confidence and self-love.

AFFIRMATIONS

I am a strong, independent black women.

*

I am the creator of my life.

* *

I can overcome anything.

* * *

I am a force to be reckoned with.

* *

Coarse or fine. Long or short - my hair tells a beautiful story that others have the privilege of bearing witness to.

*

I only speak good things about myself to all, including myself.

* *

I am deserving of kind, gentle, and genuine love.

Every day is a new opportunity to show that I am unstoppable.

* * *

Greatness lives in me.

* *

Everyone around me is a source of inspiration.

*

Success is written into my destiny - no man, woman, or any other hurdles will ever change this.

* *

I focus my time and attention on sowing and tending to the seeds that will bear an abundance of fruit in my life.

* * *

My complexion is as it should be. Exquisite in every way.

* *

Every day I discover something new that I love about myself.

*

I am becoming the woman I have envisioned.

What I have to share with the world is worthy of an audience of many.

* *

I speak with confidence despite any nervousness or doubt.

* * *

I share my perspective with the understanding that I have the power to speak into the greatness of other black women.

* *

No longer will my beauty be subject to the opinions of others; I am choosing to be my own beauty standard.

*

I belong here. I am wanted. I matter.

* *

Every day I choose me.

* * *

Life may throw me lemons, but I'll cover them in resin and show the world just how beautiful yellow is against my skin tone.

* *

Abundance is lovingly webbed into the essence of who I am.

I am my biggest priority.

*

I set healthy boundaries to ensure that I am never overwhelmed.

* *

Others may misconstrue my passion and label it as the "angry black woman," yet I will continue to be bold in spirit and strong in mind because my voice and my story matter.

* * *

I cannot be stopped.

* *

Unconditional love is my birthright.

*

My future is too good to let the preconceived notions of my skin hold me back. I am changing the status quo for the benefit of my freedom, joy, and finances.

* *

I am rich in love, joy, laughter, and hope; I have an abundant mindset.

* * *

I am radiant.

Money flows to me like a river.

* *

I am taking responsibility for the prosperity of my life. I am making active decisions about my future, and I am enjoying every part of seeking my own revelation.

*

My unique qualities are my superpower.

* *

Every day in every way I am becoming healthier.

* * *

I treat my body as the sacred gift that it is.

* *

I reject poor conditions of thought such as fear, envy, and doubt.

*

As I embark on the journey of healing, I am breaking generational curses and speaking life into my lineage as I commit to the liberation of myself and the women that come after me.

I am diligent in nurturing my soul with love, goodness, and grace.

* *

I eat good food, I nourish my hair, I accept kisses from the sun, and I have restful sleep.

* * *

I readily forgive myself and others.

* *

I appreciate the woman I am, and I am falling in love with myself more every day.

*

I use difficult experiences as a chance to grow and learn.

* *

At the intersection of my blackness and my womanhood is someone who is strong enough to be vulnerable.

* * *

I am always more than enough.

* *

I am an effortlessly gorgeous black woman. No ifs, and's or buts.

My boldness will break open doors of opportunity. My boldness will destroy the chains of preconceived notions and bring down walls of doubt.

*

Pursuing an abundance of self-love is where the adventure is.

* *

Society's everchanging definition of what a black woman should be will not bind me into apologizing for who I am.

* * *

I am patient with myself through my healing journey, and I ebb and flow with the tide.

* *

I am in awe of my ability to become all that I set my mind to.

*

I set my own standards of who I should be, according to the life that I desire for myself.

* *

I am quick to lift others around me.

* * *

I am committed to living my life the way I design it.

I am living intentionally. My future self is grateful for the decisions I am making now.

* *

I release any and all of my trauma, pain, and grief.

*

I am surrounded by love and tranquility, and I shall live in love and tranquility.

* *

I am healthy and whole. My worth is constant and unchanging.

* * *

I am a valuable asset to those around me.

* *

I am grateful for my body, and I love and accept every inch of it.

*

I choose to thrive and live a full and whole life.

* *

I am releasing whatever does not contribute to a space of wealth, health, and love.

I take back the power I once gave negative thoughts; No longer do they have a hold on my self-belief.

* * *

I am a magnet for money.

* *

I give myself the space to evolve, grow and learn.

*

I am ready to step into my destiny and I embrace every setback.

* *

Every day I am creating space for success.

* * *

I choose to surround myself with people who love me, seek to understand me, and accept me for who I am.

* *

I celebrate every success - big or small.

*

I possess the power to drastically change my circumstances.

* *

I lovingly accept all of my imperfections.

Mistakes - past, present, and future – do not define me. My character does.

* * *

I am a masterpiece; A canvas already painted that depicts a wonderful and unique story.

* *

I've got this. Now is my time to shine.

*

I can do it, so **watch me.**

JOURNAL

www.ingramcontent.com/pod-product-compliance
Lightning Source LLC
Chambersburg PA
CBHW021453070526
44577CB00002B/384